Andressa Silva Tavares
José F.Ribeiro
Sabrina M.R.Amorim

The pathophysiology of the placenta in diabetic pregnant women

Andressa Silva Tavares
José F.Ribeiro
Sabrina M.R.Amorim

The pathophysiology of the placenta in diabetic pregnant women

Clinical and perinatal impacts

ScienciaScripts

Imprint

Cover image: www.ingimage.com

This book is a translation from the original published under ISBN 978-613-9-73628-7.

Publisher:
Sciencia Scripts
is a trademark of
Dodo Books Indian Ocean Ltd. and OmniScriptum S.R.L publishing group

120 High Road, East Finchley, London, N2 9ED, United Kingdom
Str. Armeneasca 28/1, office 1, Chisinau MD-2012, Republic of Moldova, Europe
Printed at: see last page
ISBN: 978-620-7-87190-2

I dedicate this work to my parents, Raimundo Tavares Sobrinho and Lilian Guimarães Silva, for all their patience and dedication, for teaching me the values that I will carry with me as a professional.

ACKNOWLEDGEMENTS

To God, first and foremost, for guiding my steps and giving me the strength to overcome every obstacle during these years of study and to remain resilient throughout my career.

To my parents, Raimundo and Lilian, for giving me all the support I needed, for standing by me in every decision and always believing in my potential.

To my boyfriend Kássio, for encouraging me to achieve my goals and for understanding my absences. Thank you for all your affection

To my friends, especially Deise, Camila and Whesley, for always being there for me and giving me all the support I needed. Thank you for being essential in my journey as a professional and as a person.

To my friends Clarice and Jeffersson for helping me whenever I needed it. Thank you for all your support.

To the State University of Piauí, which provided me with human resources, a physical-academic and economic structure. For showing me much more than technical scientific knowledge, enhancing my personal development.

To my supervisor, Professor Ribeiro, for his patience, generosity and for sparing no effort in encouraging me to research.

To my patients, who were the foundation for my learning and taught me more than scientific content.

Finally, I would like to thank all those who, near or far, have been fundamental to my education.

To God, who created us and was creative in this task. His breath of life has sustained me and given me the courage to question realities and always propose a new world of possibilities.

SUMMARY

Gestational diabetes mellitus is an intolerance to glucose, first diagnosed during the second or third trimester of pregnancy, which may or may not persist after delivery. As gestational age advances, the size of the placenta increases. There is an increase in the levels of pregnancy-associated hormones such as oestrogen, progesterone, cortisol and placental lactogen in the maternal circulation accompanied by a growing insulin resistance usually beginning between 20 and 24 weeks of gestation. The aim of this study was to analyse the published scientific literature on the functional and morphological changes to the placenta in diabetic pregnant women, as well as their maternal and fetal complications. The PICO strategy was used to construct the search methodology. The guiding question according to the strategy was: What are the main pathophysiological changes in the placenta of pregnant women with diabetes mellitus? Based on the structured question, a consultation was carried out with the Health Sciences Descriptors (DeCS), where the descriptors that supported the search were identified on the Virtual Health Library (VHL) portal. When the search strategies were carried out on the journal portals, 333 studies were identified. After applying the inclusion and exclusion criteria, 26 articles were found. The database with the highest number of publications was Medline with 25 articles. All the articles were published in English. The year with the highest number of publications was 2014 with 11 articles. The articles were grouped according to similarities in content, from which five thematic categories emerged: The morphology of the diabetic placenta, alterations in the gene expression of Extracellular Matrix molecules, Transplacental distribution of anaesthetics in the pre-delivery period in diabetic pregnant women, Alterations in the expression of Leptin in diabetic pregnant women , the vascularisation of the diabetic placenta and maternal-fetal complications arising from gestational Diabetes mellitus. It was possible to observe a scarcity of publications on the subject under study, all of which were international. It is believed that national studies could enhance the literature and thus add knowledge and improve care for this group.

Descriptors: Placenta. Gestational diabetes. Complications.

CONTENTS

CHAPTER 1 6

CHAPTER 2 10

CHAPTER 3 14

CHAPTER 4 43

CHAPTER 5 45

CHAPTER 1

Initial considerations

Gestational diabetes mellitus (GDM) is considered to be one of the most frequent obstetric dysfunctions that occur during pregnancy, triggered by impaired maternal insulin secretion in relation to the demand before pregnancy, as well as temporary metabolic stressors imposed by the placenta, and ultimately results in hyperglycaemia of varying severity.(ANTUNES et.al., 2015).

During a healthy pregnancy, the increase in placental hormones, including prolactin and human placental lactogen, leads to an increase in insulin secretion. In contrast, women with gestational diabetes have relatively reduced levels of insulin secretion resulting in higher maternal glucose levels. Increased glycaemia in the pre- and peri-partum period is one of the main causes of foetal complications (KIM, 2014).

Insulin resistance comes from the combination of increased maternal adiposity and placental production of diabetogenic hormones, including growth hormone, cortisol, placental lactogenic hormone and progesterone. It can be seen that hyperglycaemia may be present during the period of foetal organogenesis, substantially increasing the chance of congenital malformations (CATALANO et al., 2014 a).

The placenta plays a fundamental role in maintaining pregnancy and foetal growth. Its morphogenesis and development can be compromised by high plasma glucose levels, altering the gene expression of its molecules (GIACHINI et al., 2014).

It is connected to the foetus by an umbilical vein and two umbilical arteries that form part of the umbilical cord. The umbilical vein carries arterialised blood from the placenta and the arteries carry venous blood to the placenta. In cases of gestational diabetes, there is excessive coiling of this cord, seriously damaging foetal circulation (HERRERA; DESOYE, 2016).

The placenta produces all kinds of cytokines, including tumour necrosis factor alpha (TNF-a), resistin and leptin, which are produced by adipose tissue. These hormones can lead to insulin resistance, contributing to the development of gestational diabetes (HE et al., 2016). A state of persistent hyperglycaemia caused by GDM leads to various changes in the body, including changes in the pattern of synthesis and/or release of various substances, such as hormones, cytokines or growth factors (STANEK, 2017).

GDM is a considerable risk factor for foetal macrosomia, as it causes increased glucose administration to the foetus, which consequently leads to premature maturation of pancreatic insulin secretion and subsequent hyperinsulinaemia, which, together with excessive glucose availability, results in excessive foetal growth (CATALANO; MOUZON, 2015).

In diabetic pregnancies there is a wide range of disturbances in lipid metabolism, where maternal lipids are strong determinants of foetal growth in pregnancies. Although lipids cross the placenta with some difficulty, changes in placental function contribute to an increase in the transfer of maternal lipids to the foetus in conditions of hyperlipidaemia (VRIES et al., 2014).

Women with a history of gestational diabetes mellitus are at greater risk of glucose intolerant states after giving birth, including gestational diabetes in future pregnancies. This is because placental and foetal factors impose stresses on maternal metabolism that have lasting effects due to these changes in fat mass distribution. The magnitude of this "permanent" weight gain attributed to pregnancy is directly related to the degree of gestational weight gain and persists over a decade after giving birth (ZHANG et al., 2015).

The effects of GDM can be seen in the disturbance of energy homeostasis in placental expression of genes that regulate the size, function and endocrine sensitivity of the placenta. Diabetes, regardless of whether it has good or poor metabolic control, modifies the processes of vasculogenesis and angiogenesis, altering vascular morphology, which implies that there are consequences for the foetus (MARTINO et al., 2016).

1.1 Guiding question

What are the main pathophysiological changes that occur in the placenta of pregnant women with Diabetes Mellitus?

1.2 Aim of the study

To analyse the functional and morphological changes in the placenta of diabetic pregnant women, as well as their maternal-fetal complications.

1.3 Justification and relevance

The topic was chosen because of the perception of the range of alterations to the placenta in pregnant women caused by diabetes mellitus, in view of the growing number of women who develop this pathology.

As a result, questions arose about what the literature has to offer on this subject.

Given this panorama, the study is relevant due to the scarcity of national publications on this subject, enhancing the knowledge of health professionals, as well as pregnant women who experience DM.

Furthermore, they can subsidise the production of information on the subject, triggering health education actions and contributing to the formulation of strategies to reduce gestational diabetes and improve the quality of care provided to patients.

For the scientific group, the study is very important and could be used as a basis for future research on the same subject.

CHAPTER 2

Methodology

2.1 Type of study

This is an integrative literature review with a qualitative approach in order to obtain information on the main functional and morphological alterations of the placenta in pregnant women with gestational diabetes.

The term integrative comes from the relationship between opinions, concepts or ideas from the research used in the method, a point that ratifies the potential for building science. It also enables the researcher to get closer to the problem they want to assess, drawing up an overview of their scientific output in order to learn about the evolution of the subject over time and thus visualise possible research opportunities (GALVÃO; SAWADA; TREVISAN, 2004).

According to Gil (2002), bibliographical research is carried out using data or information that has already been worked on and recorded by other researchers who propose the construction of theories and conceptual frameworks using the deductive method.

The main advantage of bibliographical research lies in the fact that it allows the researcher to cover a much wider range of phenomena than could be researched directly. This benefit becomes particularly important when the research problem requires data that is widely dispersed over space (Gil, 2002).

Most bibliographical research can be defined as exploratory studies, which aim to provide greater familiarity with the problem in order to make it more explicit and build hypotheses (Gil, 2002).

2.2 Procedures and methods

In order to draw up this integrative review, we went through six stages, which are set out in the table below.

Chart 1. Stages for drawing up an integrative literature review. Teresina, Piauí, 2017.

1ST STAGE	Identification of the topic and research question
2° STAGE	Establishment of criteria for inclusion and exclusion of studies
3RD STAGE	Definition of the information to be extracted from the selected studies
4THETAPA	Evaluation of the studies included in the integrative review
5TH STAGE	Interpreting the results
6TH STAGE	Presentation of the review

Source: MENDES; SILVEIRA; GALVÃO, 2008.

The PICO strategy was used in this study, where P - Patient or problem ;I - Intervention; C - Control or comparison group ;O - outcome (results).

For this study, the following were considered: P - diabetic pregnant women; I - not applicable to the study; C - placenta of diabetic and non-diabetic pregnant women; O - changes in the placenta of diabetic pregnant women.

The inclusion criteria were articles available in full text during the last four years, in national and international scientific journals, written in Portuguese and English and addressing the theme. Articles that were repeated, not found in full or that did not answer the guiding question were excluded from this study.

The search for articles was carried out using the Health Sciences Descriptors (DECS), which were used: Placenta; Gestational diabetes; Complications.

Data was collected online in November 2017 using an instrument previously prepared in Microsoft Office Excel 2013, which contained the following variables: title of the journal, title of the article, academic background of the 1st author, year of publication and type of study (Appendix).

After identifying, locating and obtaining the works, the material was read. Initially, exploratory reading was carried out, which is a reading of the bibliographic material with the aim of ascertaining the extent to which the work consulted is of interest to the research (Gil, 2002).

This was followed by selection, i.e. selective reading, where the material that was of real interest to the research was determined on the basis of the research objectives. Analytical reading was carried out on the basis of the selected texts in order to organise and summarise the information (Gil, 2002).

Interpretative reading was the last stage in the process of reading bibliographic sources. According to Gil (2002), it is the most complex, since its aim is to relate what the author says to the problem for which a solution is proposed.

CHAPTER 3

Results and discussion

3.1 Characterisation of the studies

Flowchart 1: Characterisation of the studies

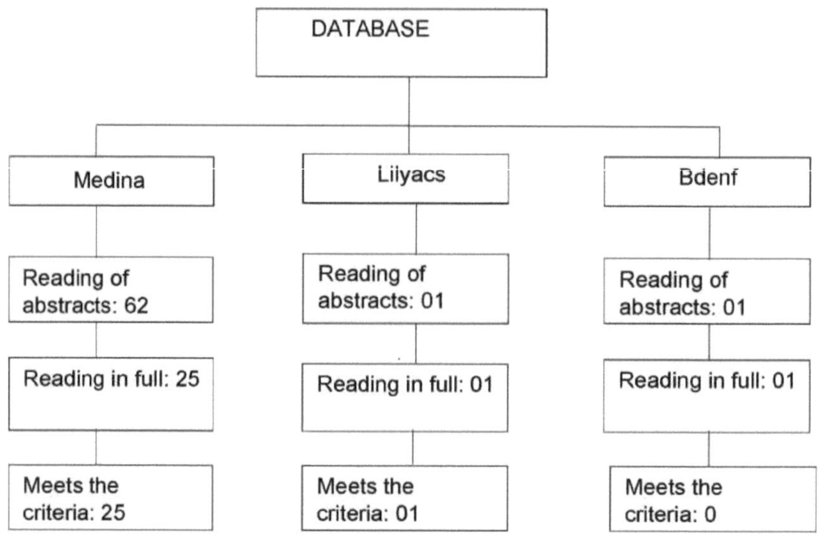

Source: Prepared by the author, 2017.

When the search strategies were applied to the journal portals according to the descriptors: Placenta; Gestational Diabetes and Complications, 333 articles were found. In the Medline portal, 318 articles were found and, after applying the inclusion criteria, 62 remained. Of these, 37 did not cover the subject of the study, and 25 articles were pre-selected.

On the Lilacs portal, 14 articles were found and, after applying the inclusion criteria, only one remained, which was included.

One article was found on the Bdenf portal, which did not have the pre-established theme. Thus, after applying the inclusion and exclusion criteria associated with the reading, 63 pre-selected articles were found. After detailed reading, it was noted that 37 did not contain information on the established theme, and the study sample consisted of 26 articles.

Based on the search carried out for this study, it was observed that different types of study have been published in health journals by authors from different backgrounds, as can be seen in Chart 2.

Table 2. Distribution of the sample according to journal, type of study and academic background of the 1st author. Teresina, Piauí, 2017.

JOURNAL OF PUBLICATION	TYPE OF STUDY	ACADEMIC BACKGROUND OF THE 1ST AUTHOR
British Journal of Clinical Pharmacology	Field research	Pharmacist
Molecular Nutrition & Food Research	Field research	Biochemistry
Acta Obstet Gynecol Scand	Field research	Medical
International journal of obesity	Field research	Doctor
Diabetic medicine :a journal of the British Diabetic Association	Literature review	Doctor
Am J Obstet Gynecol	Field research	Doctor
Diabetology 59	Bibliographical review	Doctor

Obes Silver Spring Md	Field research	Doctor
Journal of Anatomy	Field research	Biomedical
BMJ Open	Field research	Doctor
Journal of Perinatal Medicine	Field research	Doctor
Postgraduate Medical Journal	Field research	Doctor
Molecular Hormone Biology and Clinical Investigation	Literature review	Biochemist
Journal of Obstetrics and Gynaecology Research	Field research	Doctor
Ann Nutr Metab	Literature review	Doctor
Diabetic medicine : a journal of the British Diabetic Association	Field research	Doctor
Ann Nutr Metab	Field research	Doctor
American journal of obstetrics and gynecology	Field research	Doctor
Reproductive Sciences	Field research	Doctor
American Journal of Epidemiology	Field research	Doctor
Cell Physiol Biochem	Field research	Doctor
Pathology - Research and Practice	Field research	Doctor
The Journal of Clinical Endocrinology and Metabolism	Field research	Doctor
Pios One	Field research	Doctor
Journal of Perinatal Medicine	Field research	Doctor

Prostaglandins Leukot Essent Fatty Acids	Field research	Doctor

The journal with the highest number of publications on the subject was Ann Nutr Metab with 02 articles and the type of study that stood out was field research with a total of 22 articles. With regard to the academic background of the first author, there was a predominance of medical professionals with 22 articles.

Table 3 shows the analysis of the articles in terms of title and year of publication.

Table 3. Number of studies according to article title and year of publication.Teresina,Piauí,2017.

ARTICLE TITLE	YEAR OF PUBLICATION
Influence of gestational diabetes on the stereoselective pharmacokinetics and placental distribution of metoprolol and its metabolites in parturients	2015
Placental dysfunction is associated with altered microRNA expression in pregnant women with low folate status	2017
Assessment of first-trimester thymus size and correlation with maternal diseases and foetal outcome	2016
Maternal obesity and metabolic	2015

risk to the offspring: why lifestyle interventions may not have achieved the desired outcomes	
Inadequate weight gain in overweight and obese pregnancy women: what is the effect on fetal growth?	2014
Trying to understand gestational diabetes	2014
The Fetal Glucose Steal: An Underappreciated Phenomenon in Diabetic Pregnancy.	2016
The long-term impact of intrauterine growth restriction in a diverse U.S. cohort of children: the EPOCH study	2014
Maternal Diabetes Affects Specific Extracellular Matrix Components during Placentation	2014
Genetics of Glucose regulation in Gestation and Growth (Gen3G): a prospective prebirth cohort of mother- child pairs in Sherbrooke,	2016
Maternal serum placental growth factor and fetal SGA in pregnancy complicated by type	2014

1 diabetes mellitus.	
The impact of gestational weight gain in different trimesters of pregnancy on glucose challenge test and gestational diabetes	2016
Maternal and foetal lipid metabolism under normal and gestational diabetic conditions.	2016
Decidual arteriolopathy with or without associated hypertension modifies the underlying histomorphology in placentas from diabetic mothers	2017
Gestational Diabetes Mellitus and Macrosomics: A Literature Review	2015
Maternal outcomes and follow-up after gestational diabetes mellitus	2014
Placental Fatty Acid Transfer: A Key Factor in Fetal Growth	2014
Maternal Obesity and Gestational Diabetes are Associated with Placental Leptin DNA Methylation	2014
Early Pregnancy Maternal Lipid Profiles and the Risk of	2015

Gestational Diabetes Mellitus Stratified for Body Mass Index	
Placental Weight and Male Genital Anomalies: A Nationwide Danish Cohort Study	2016
Distinct DNA Methylomes of Human Placentas Between Pre-Eclampsia and Gestational Diabetes Mellitus	2014
Placental findings associated with maternal obesity at early pregnancy	2016
Maternal Body Weight and Gestational Diabetes Differentially Influence Placental and Pregnancy Outcomes	2016
Synthetic PreImplantation Factor (PIF) prevents foetal loss by modulating LPS induced inflammatory response	2017
Relation of placental diagnosis in stillbirth to fetal maceration and gestational age at delivery	2014
Association between polyunsaturated fatty acid concentrations in maternal	2014
plasma phospholipids during pregnancy and offspring	

adiposity at age 7: the MEFAB cohort	

Source: direct collection

Analysing the articles in the table above, it can be seen that all the studies are in English, which clearly shows the need for national publications. Regarding the year of publication, 2014 prevailed with 11 articles and 2016 with 8 articles.

3.2 Categorisation of studies

3.2.1 The morphology of the diabetic placenta

According to Catalano et al. (2014a) the human placenta plays a central role in regulating foetal growth, establishing a maximum size that can be linked to a given placental size. Accurate examination of the placenta can provide insights into the intrauterine environment before birth.

The growth of the foetus is mainly influenced by the weight and functional value of the placenta. In bivitelline twins, the heavier foetus corresponds to the heavier placenta. The ability of the foetus to grow and mature in the womb is related to the placenta's ability to offer nutrients to the foetus. However, it is often the most neglected organ in the body (ARENDT et al., 2016).

The formation of the human placenta takes place when extravillous cytotrophoblasts invade the superficial part of the uterus, in the direction of the spiral arteries, replacing the maternal endothelial cells and the arterial smooth muscle tunic, making it insensitive to vasoactive elements, which allows perfusion of the intervillous chamber (BORGELT et al., 2016).

This process involves the degradation of enzymes that facilitate uterine revascularisation. The maternal inflammatory response at the time of placental formation is essential in understanding placental changes, and it is fundamental to realise that the adequacy of placental function comes from this mechanism, among other factors (CRUME et.al, 2014).

Placental size is a manifestation that accompanies foetal growth and has no independent clinical significance, given the positive correlation between foetal weight and placental weight. The regular increase in placental weight is closely related to the continuous progress of the internal structuring of the villous tree. There is also an increase in the number of foetal vessels and a sinusoidal transformation of capillaries into branches and villi (GIACHINI et al., 2014).

The size of the diabetic placenta is notable for its large volume, especially when the diabetes is of recent origin or poorly controlled. Placental thickness correlates with gestational age, where normal growth in thickness is around 1mm per week. Placentomegaly, on the other hand, refers to an abnormally thickened placenta, greater than 40 mm (GUTAJ et al., 2014).

Placentas from mothers with GDM and poor glycaemic control show villous oedema, fibrin deposits in the syncytiotrophoblast and hyperplasia of the cytotrophoblast, impairing feto-placental haemodynamics, where oxygen saturation is significantly reduced in the umbilical vein in these cases (HE et al., 2016).

In general, the greater the macrosomia of the foetus, the greater the size of the placenta. The increase in weight is not due to the accumulation of water, but due to the increase in cellular content, especially in placentas with class A diabetes. On the other hand, in diabetic pregnant women without vasculopathy, the placentas are larger, heavier, with hyperplasia of cells, due to the increase in the speed of cell division, which occurs before the 36th week (HERRERA; DESOYE, 2016).

Examination of the placenta provides information about the intrauterine environment. It can be seen that a poor intrauterine environment is a risk factor for the development of hypertension and diabetes in adulthood (GUTAJ et al., 2014).

According to Arendt et al. (2016) placental weight is significantly higher in class B+C diabetic pregnant women compared to class D+R, an indication that placental weight in these patients is influenced by the duration and severity of the vascular complications of diabetes.

When comparing the existence of placental degenerative lesions, such as fibrinoid necrosis or chorangiosis, in normal pregnancies and those with GDM, they are seen more frequently in the latter. At the same time, some indicators of chronic foetal hypoxia are also observed in pregnant women with this disease, such as an increase in the number of nucleated red blood cells and more immature villi (BORGELT et al., 2016).

These, together with fibrinoid necrosis, make gas exchange difficult, as they increase the distance between the intervillous space, where maternal blood circulates, and the foetal capillaries. Therefore, in an attempt to compensate for the deficient diffusion of oxygen, there is an increase in the growth of the villi to increase the surface area for exchange and also an increase in angiogenesis, which in many cases leads to an increased placental weight (GUTAJ et al., 2014).

Due to the dependence of the connection between the placenta and the foetus, altered placental function predicts different patterns of pregnancy outcomes and establishes the evolution of foetal injury, which makes the foetus more prone to foetal hypoxia and therefore interferes with maternal-foetal exchange mechanisms and the production of amniotic fluid. In addition, placental gigantism is associated with higher perinatal mortality (STANEK, 2017).

3.2.2 Changes in gene expression of Extracellular Matrix molecules

The extracellular matrix (ECM) is the grouping of intercellular elements and corresponds to the complex of macromolecules constituting a variety of proteins and versatile polysaccharides arranged in a network associated with the cell surface (GIACHINI et al., 2014).

ECM is necessary for many specialised cell functions and consists of various associations of molecules, such as collagens, elastin, glycosaminoglycans and proteoglycans, which give rise to long fibres and multi-adhesive proteins (KAMANA; SHAKYA; ZHANG, 2015).

An important discovery was the detection of alterations in the gene expression of type I collagen and also in the deposition of collagens and proteoglycans in the decidua of diabetic pregnant women. These molecular changes in the ECM are capable of modifying the molecular dialogue between the embryo and the mother, impairing embryonic development (ABI-ABIB et al., 2014).

Proper foetal growth and development depend on adequate placental function. Given that diabetes affects placentation, its effects on the expression, organisation and alteration of extracellular matrix components in various organs, as well as tissue remodelling and fibrosis, can be verified (CATALANO, 2014b).

Considering that high plasma glucose levels modify the gene expression of ECM molecules in cells, it can be inferred that its composition plays a role during embryo implantation and placentation. Thus, it can be observed that ECM molecules are differentially expressed in the various compartments of the placenta, suggesting that specific microenvironments are created within it (LESSEUR et.al,2014).

It is worth noting that ECM molecules are modulated during placental development and diabetes has a direct impact on the distribution and expression of some molecules, such as fibronectin (GUILLEMETTE et al., 2016).

Diabetes affects the expression of fibronectin, which is present in placentas of diabetic pregnant women and is found in the umbilical cord mesenchyme and extracellular matrix. This molecule has been associated with the degree of tissue maturation and its high levels indicate immature chorionic villi in human placentas (MARTINO et al., 2016).

According to Li et al. (2015) the deposition of ECM molecules in the tissues of diabetic pregnant women has been correlated with increased expression of transforming growth factor beta, an inducer of fibronectin production in the glomeruli of diabetic pregnant women.

Fibronectin deposition, unlike other molecules, is particularly affected by diabetes. The altered deposition of extracellular matrix molecules can modify the placental microenvironment, leading to developmental abnormalities in the placenta of diabetic pregnant women (LIU et.al, 2014).

In short, during placental development, specific ECM molecules are secreted in various parts of the placenta. In addition, the deposition of some of these molecules is modulated by the pregnancy itself, depending on the degree of placental maturity (LIU et al., 2014).

The changes caused by diabetes in the decidua and its ECM may contribute significantly to the higher incidence of miscarriages and malformations in diabetic pregnancies. It is therefore inferred that these changes in the ECM caused by gestational diabetes mellitus are also involved in teratogenicity (VRIES et al., 2014).

3.2.3 Transplacental distribution of anaesthetics in the pre-delivery period in diabetic pregnant women

Anaesthesia in pregnant patients involves a number of situations that must be analysed carefully before it is offered. In addition to the exposure of the foetus to anaesthesia and the possible toxicity of the agents to be used, the gestational period, each drug and the doses to be used must be taken into account (ANTUNES et al., 2015).

Diabetes mellitus has the ability to alter pharmacokinetics by various mechanisms, including a change in intestinal absorption, distribution and elimination of clinically used drugs, **which** can contribute to foetal hypoxia and increased foetal and neonatal morbidity associated with this pathology. Transplacental drug distribution generally occurs by passive diffusion (STANEK, 2017).

Various drugs are transported across the placenta by simple diffusion, without energy expenditure, depending on the concentration of the free drug, the ratio and the extent of the placental exchange barrier. This transport favours the passage of lipophilic agents, and due to their physical and chemical characteristics, practically all anaesthetic agents cross the placental barrier (LARQUÉ et al., 2014).

The binding of drugs to plasma proteins may be altered in this condition, due to the high concentration of free fatty acids and glycosylated proteins, causing changes in the distribution and elimination of substrates (SINGH; SINGH, 2015).

In order to provide quality obstetric anaesthetic care, labour and the surgical anaesthetic procedure must be conducted on the basis of knowledge of pregnancy physiology. Medicines manipulated in clinical practice follow stages of absorption, distribution, metabolism and elimination. However, each of these stages is often modified by the influence of a disease, such as gestational diabetes mellitus (ZHANG et al., 2015).

Local anaesthetics rapidly cross the placental barrier and the repercussions on the neonate depend on the amount that crosses this barrier, which is determined by the pharmacokinetics of the drug in the mother, the foetus and the placenta. The placenta is a metabolic organ and therefore respects the principles of a metabolic barrier. (GUTAJ et al., 2014).

The placentas of pregnant women with GDM have small and numerous terminal villi, resulting in a significant increase in the extent of the maternal-fetal exchange surface. In addition, the capillarisation index is lower and these changes in placentation can directly influence the rate of transplacental transfer of drugs used during pregnancy (GUILLEMETTE et al., 2016).

The epidural space has negative pressure, fatty tissue and rich vascularisation, making it possible for anaesthetic drugs injected into this space to be rapidly absorbed. However, in diabetic pregnant women, the plasma concentrations of these anaesthetics are increased, as GDM inhibits the metabolisation of these drugs by partially blocking the biotransformation of the original drug (DESOYE; NOLAN, 2016).

In this way, these changes lead to responses such as oxidative stress, which is responsible for the pathophysiological complications caused by diabetes mellitus that hinder the normal development of pregnancy associated with the molecular mechanism of decreased insulin biosynthesis and secretion, being the main etiology of glucose toxicity (CATALANO; MOUZON, 2015).

It is valid to consider that pregnancy is a period that tends towards a growing increase in insulin resistance from the beginning of the second half of the pregnancy until the end of the third trimester, being intensified in pregnant women who have GDM. This state regresses after labour, as placental hormones play the main role in the genesis of insulin resistance (SIMONE et al., 2017).

3.2.4 Changes in Leptin expression in diabetic pregnant women

Pregnancy is a period marked by profound changes in a woman's metabolic and hormonal state. The ability to regulate the balance of nutrients during this period is crucial for both mother and foetus. Insulin is one of the key regulators of metabolism and changes in insulin sensitivity and its ability to control blood glucose levels, body fat and protein levels during pregnancy are mainly present in the later stages of gestation (CRUME et.al., 2014).

In the foetus, the intrauterine development of adipose tissue takes place in two phases: one of maturation, which occurs predominantly in the second trimester, and one of accumulation, which takes place in the third trimester. The placenta, a metabolically active organ that regulates the intrauterine environment, is a substantial source of leptin during pregnancy, with levels of this hormone increasing significantly, regardless of Body Mass Index (BMI), and decreasing slightly after delivery (HANTOUSHZADEH et al., 2016).

Diabetes mellitus in pregnant women causes generalised changes in the expression of placental genes, creating a lipotoxic placental environment. During pregnancy, leptin is produced by the placenta where it has pleiotropic functions, including growth regulation and nutrient exchange. Thus, maternal obesity caused by DM affects placental resistance to leptin, causing a reduction in LEP gene expression. (GUTAJ et al., 2014).

Leptin is an adipokine, i.e. a peptide hormone produced by adipose tissue encoded by the LEP gene and functions as part of a signalling pathway that can inhibit food intake and/or regulate energy expenditure to maintain fat mass constancy (ROMANOWSKI et al., 2015).

This adipokine is released into the circulation at levels proportional to lipid reserves and acts on the brain and other tissues, participating in a negative feedback mechanism related to the maintenance of energy homeostasis (LESSEUR et al., 2014).

[a]In pregnant women, due to the increase in fat mass and the presence of the placenta, the amount of maternal leptin increases 2 to 3 times above the concentration of non-pregnant women, with the peak occurring on average from the 28th week of pregnancy (ZHANG et al., 2015).

Leptin acts as a foetal and newborn growth factor and its concentration correlates with gestational age, a fact that is consistent with the pattern of adipose tissue development and the accumulation of fat mass by the foetus during pregnancy (ABI-ABIB et al., 2014).

During pregnancy, leptin regulates placental development, nutrient transfer, angiogenesis, lung maturation and trophoblast invasion. Thus, one of the functions of leptin during pregnancy is to mobilise the mother's lipid reserves and increase the availability and placental transfer of lipid substrates to the foetus (CATALANO, 2014 b).

Both insulin and hypoxia are stimuli of the leptin gene, where an increase in the production of this gene causes placental insufficiency, suggesting that this may be an index of foetal stress, inflammatory response and placental dysfunction. (BAKER et al., 2017).

Leptin also appears to have an autocrine role in the placenta, and abnormal trophoblastic invasion or proliferation is associated with atypical release of leptin, indicating that it may be directly involved in placental growth. (LESSEUR et al., 2014).

Plasma concentrations of leptin are elevated in the umbilical cord blood of children born to obese mothers with gestational diabetes. Although foetal hyperleptinaemia may contribute to the induction of leptin resistance by chronic activation of leptin receptors in the foetus, it is not known whether hypothalamic leptin targets respond before birth or whether neonatal leptin resistance leads to adverse long-term consequences (MARTINO et al., 2016).

The increase in circulating leptin in cord blood leads to potential adiposity performance in the newborn and impaired immune responses, as well as being related to the maturation of the hypothalamus (ROMANOWSKI et al., 2015).

During normal pregnancy, placental production of leptin provides a hyperleptinemic state that is compensated for by hypothalamic resistance to leptin, which is necessary to increase food intake. Furthermore, as pregnancy progresses, progressive insulin resistance occurs, mediated in part by increased adiposity and placental hormones (VRIES et al., 2014).

In GDM, pregnancy-induced insulin resistance generally occurs in relation to the state of chronic insulin resistance that is regularly associated with obesity. Thus, studies show that GDM acts as a partial mediator of the effects of maternal obesity on the epigenetic control of placental LEP DNA methylation. (LESSEUR et al., 2014).

It can therefore be inferred that GDM is associated with an increase in placental leptin expression and an increase in the production of inflammatory cytokines (TNF-a and IL-6). Increased leptin concentrations may therefore represent a pro-inflammatory state and insulin resistance (BAKER et al., 2017).

3.2.5 The vascularisation of the diabetic placenta

The placenta is a temporary organ that develops continuously only during pregnancy. It separates maternal and foetal blood circulation and ensures the passage of all nutrients and oxygen from the mother to the foetus, as well as the excretion of the products of the latter's metabolism. In addition, it does not allow them to come into direct contact, acting as a facilitator of the necessary exchanges between the two (CRUME et al., 2014).

Therefore, as the placenta acts as an interface, it is understandable that it is concomitantly exposed to maternal and foetal molecules and is affected by them. On the other hand, it is itself an endocrine organ and producer of substances that exert their action on the mother and foetus independently (HERRERA; DESOYE, 2016).

In GDM there is structural and functional immaturity of the placenta in relation to gestational age, which includes increased size of the terminal villus, an oedematous appearance, decreased vascularisation and formation of the vascular-syncytial membrane, residual cytotrophoblast and increased Hofbauer cells (CRUME etal ., 2014). The Placental morphological changes in diabetic pregnant women are similar to those in insulin-dependent patients, but to a lesser extent. These changes predict that maternal illness can produce a range of alterations in the placental micrometabolic environment. (ZHANG et al.,2015).

The placental vascular bed is interconnected with the foetal circulatory system and placental capillaries play an indispensable role in the transfer of oxygen, nutrients and metabolites between maternal and foetal blood. As foetal development is absolutely dependent on their functional efficiency, any disorder of them can jeopardise foetal well-being (CRUME et.al, 2014).

According to Catalano et al. (2014a), GDM considerably influences the placental microvascular bed. This influence is manifested by the altered size and course of the capillaries, the altered structure of the fast stroma and the increased sprouted angiogenesis in the terminal villi. It can also be seen that there is a significant increase in capillary branching in DM placentas.

Vascularisation depends on the growth and maturation of the villi. During pregnancy, the development of the villous tree occurs basically as a result of the growth of the intermediate and terminal villi. However, in diabetes there is an increase in the number of immature intermediate villi and a smaller number of terminal villi (HERRERA; DESOYE, 2016).

In GDM, there may be changes in angiogenesis and vessel permeability, with increased maternal levels of glucose, insulin, angiogenic factors, cytokines and inflammatory mediators, which will have a direct impact on some or even all of the stages of vessel formation (STANEK, 2017).

Therefore, according to Catalano (2014 b), in a situation of DM prior to pregnancy there is a metabolic insult that will have long-term effects on placental development, whereas in GDM this insult will have a short-term effect, given that most of the gestational period took place in an environment of normoglycaemia (Figure 1).

Figure 1: The growth and development of the placenta

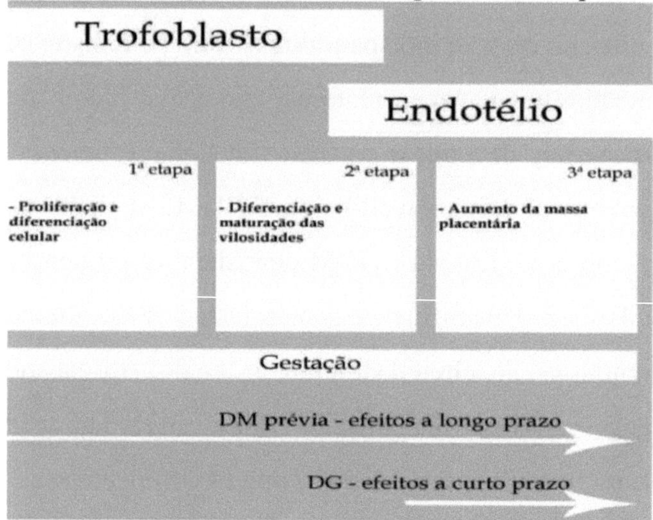

Figure 1 : The growth and development of the placenta essentially depends on three main stages, with the trophoblast playing a predominant role in the first half of pregnancy and the endothelium in the second half. The presence of diabetes prior to pregnancy has long-term effects on placental development. Gestational diabetes, on the other hand, has short-term effects.

DM = diabetes mellitus ; GD = gestational diabetes

Source: Reis, 2012.

Vasculogenesis begins around the 21st day of gestation and leads to the formation of the first primitive vessels, while angiogenesis begins later, on the 32nd day, generating extensive vascular networks due to the high branching rate of the newly formed vessels (LIU et al., 2014).

Angiogenesis also depends on oxygen concentrations in placental tissues, and hypoxia regulates receptor expression and

production of growth factors. The synthesis of new placental vessels in the first trimester, the maturation of vessels in the first and second trimesters and angiogenesis in the third trimester take place in a space of hyperglycaemia (HERRERA; DESOYE, 2016).

The visible differences in stromal cells between normal and pathological villi suggest that maternal diabetes interferes with the differentiation of stromal cells and also differs in the organisation of collagen fibrils. The loose arrangement of collagen fibrils in diabetic villi is equivalent to a decrease in the amount of collagen (LIU et al., 2014).

The foetus, in turn, reacts by overproducing insulin growth factors, which causes additional changes in the structure and growth of the placenta. (BORGELT et al., 2016).

The placenta can then be seen as a large microvascular bed, embedded in a thin layer of syncytiotrophoblast, which is bathed in maternal blood flowing from the spiral arteries. The vessels are naturally capable of responding to vasoactive agents, oxygen, growth factors, hormones, glucose and nutrients, among others. However, this capacity may be insufficient to protect the foetus in pregnancies complicated by this pathology (ZHANG et al., 2015).

All these changes make it more difficult to carry out gas exchange, since the gases have a larger diffusion surface to cross, causing a situation of chronic foetal hypoxia. Hyperglycaemia therefore affects the quality of gas exchange in the placenta and the amount of surface area available for it to take place (LIU et al., 2014).

These vascular alterations are typical of the third trimester of pregnancy, occurring essentially in the process of angiogenesis, with vasculogenesis not being affected. This causes a weakness in placental function, with greater difficulty in carrying out exchanges between mother and foetus, as the changes occur during the phase of greatest expansion of the placental mass (CRUME et al., 2014).

3.2.6 Maternal-fetal complications of gestational diabetes mellitus

Diabetes mellitus is related to certain aspects of lifestyle, such as a high-calorie, high-fat diet, smoking and a sedentary lifestyle. Pregnant women can also be affected by this disease, thus determining two different situations: either diabetes existed prior to pregnancy or it is diagnosed for the first time during the pregnancy period, becoming known as gestational diabetes (GD). (CATALANO et al., 2014 a).

In any of the above situations, there are risks and pregnant women should be carefully monitored. The risk is not only maternal, but there may also be complications for the foetus (CATALANO; MOUZON, 2015).

The placenta is an organ whose basic function is to transport nutrients and metabolites between the maternal and foetal circulations. The maternal concentration of nutrients, the permeability of the placental barrier and uterine and umbilical blood flow are all factors that can modify transport through the placenta. (CATALANO et al., 2014 a).

This organ has the ability to adjust maternal blood glucose levels within certain limits, as it can act as a buffer system for excess glucose. However, if its maximum capacity is exceeded, it is unable to prevent the passage of glucose to the foetus, with the implications that this entails. (HANTOUSHZADEH et al.,2016).

There is a high consumption of glucose by the placenta, as the uteroplacental tissue uses a high rate of this energy substrate, as well as oxygen, with almost the same consumption observed in the tissues of the central nervous system. Around half of the oxygen and 2/3 of the glucose coming from the pregnant woman's circulation is utilised by these tissues (LI et al., 2015).

Hyperglycaemia in pregnant women contributes not only to an increase in maternal insulin, but also to fetal hyperinsulinaemia, since if there are no changes in transport in the placenta, glucose crosses it due to the transplacental gradient that is established, passing into the fetal circulation and stimulating insulin production by the fetus's pancreas, with a high probability of triggering pancreatic beta cell hyperplasia (LARQUÉ et al., 2014).

In the foetus, the amount of glucose depends on the concentration provided by the umbilical vein, endogenous production by the breakdown of glycogen and synthesis by carbohydrate sources. This glucose is used for metabolism's own expenses, with the production of CO_2 and the consumption of oxygen. It can also be stored in the form of protein deposits, glycogen energy reserves and fat (KIM, 2014).

This combination of hyperinsulinaemia and hyperglycaemia results in a cascade of events that culminates in a large increase in fat deposits and an increase in protein stores, making the foetus macrosomic, which predisposes it to tocotrauma, especially shoulder dystocia. The main complication is brachial plexus injury, with homolateral motor alterations and extension of the right upper limb (KAMANA; SHAKYA; ZHANG, 2015).

The simultaneous increase in fetal glycaemia and insulinemia clearly contributes to one of the most frequently observed changes in pregnancy associated with diabetes: fetal macrosomia (DESOYE; NOLAN, 2016).

Diabetic fetopathy, which usually occurs in the second and third trimesters, causes fetal hyperinsulinemia and macrosomia, the latter defined as birth weight equal to or above 4,000 g or above the 90th percentile for gestational age (LI et al., 2015).

In addition, the existence of maternal diabetes is particularly related to an increased risk of childhood obesity and metabolic syndrome for the still developing foetus (KAMANA; SHAKYA; ZHANG, 2015).

Chronic foetal hyperinsulinaemia results in accentuated metabolic values that increase oxygen consumption and foetal hypoxaemia, which contributes to the newborn's increased mortality, metabolic acidosis, changes in iron distribution and increased erythropoiesis. It can also lead to late-onset obesity and impaired psychomotor development (DESOYE; NOLAN, 2016).

Due to a weakness in placental function, it is more difficult to carry out exchanges between mother and foetus, as the alterations occur during the phase of greatest expansion of the placental mass. As a result, there is a higher incidence of deaths in utero, foetuses with excessive weight for gestational age and prematurity, when compared to normal pregnancies and also to pregnancies with previous DM. (STANEK; BIESIADA, 2014).

Polycythaemia, another considerable complication, drives the production of catecholamines, which can result in systemic arterial hypertension and cardiac hypertrophy. As the foetus increases the number of red blood cells, the redistribution of iron causes iron deficiency in the developing organs, contributing to cardiomyopathy and alterations in neuropsychomotor development (KIM, 2014).

In addition, other perceived complications are the formation of breech, meconium production and acute fetal distress, resulting from the increased labour time. Maternal hyperglycaemia also delays the synthesis of surfactant, an effective substance for fetal lung maturation, since neonatal hyperinsulinaemia interferes with glucocorticoid levels, which are responsible for stimulating the production of surfactant itself (KIM, 2014).

In order to prevent neonatal sequelae and reduce the frequency and severity of complications, it is essential to maintain good glycaemic control, through maternal and fetal antepartum monitoring and providing pregnant women with knowledge of the maternal and fetal risks related to the disease (CATALANO; MOUZON, 2015).

Among the maternal complications resulting from GDM are an increase in pre-eclampsia (10 to 30 per cent) compared to those with normal glucose tolerance (5 to 7 per cent risk) and a higher rate of caesarean sections due to the foetus becoming macrosomic when exposed to maternal hyperglycaemia (SINGH; SINGH, 2015).

Furthermore, GDM substantially increases the chance of developing diabetes after childbirth, with a risk of approximately 40 per cent after a 10-year follow-up period. Retinopathy and nephropathy are relevant maternal complications, especially in those who already had such complications (ABI-ABIB et al., 2014).

Urinary infections can also occur, which are common in diabetic pregnancies, as well as premature labour due to excess amniotic fluid in the uterus, which can also cause an exaggerated increase in belly size and body weight (LARQUÉ et al., 2014).

Neonatal hypoglycaemia, characterised by blood glucose levels below 35mg/dl in the first 12 hours of life, is one of the most common neonatal complications in diabetic pregnancies, affecting 10 to 50% of them (ABI-ABIB et al., 2014).

The mechanisms involved in the occurrence of this abnormality are not completely defined and deserve further study. It is known, however, that chronic exposure of the foetus to the maternal hyperglycaemic state results in hyperplasia of the pancreatic islets with consequent hyperinsulinaemia and neonatal hypoglycaemia (LI et al., 2015).

The importance of good glycaemic control during pregnancy in diabetic women has been well recommended by health professionals for decades. This is because the repercussions of poor metabolic control on the foetus can be toxic and are also extremely negative for the pregnant woman, as shown in Figure 2.

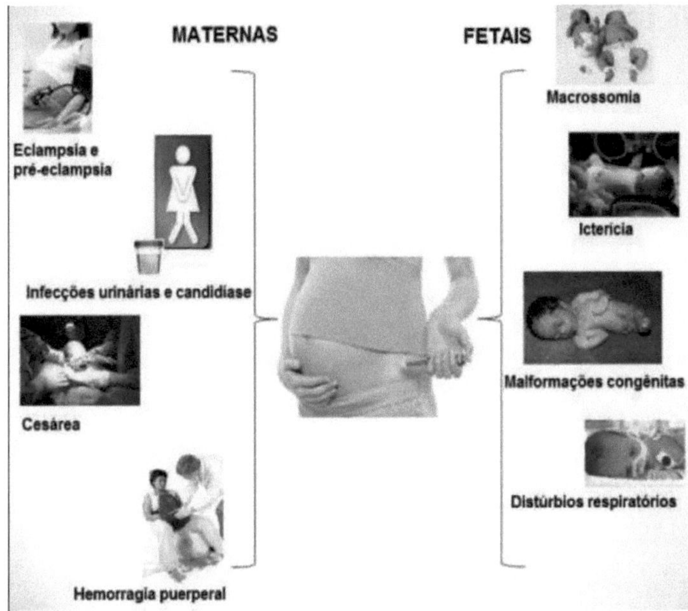

Figure 2: Complications caused by GDM.

Source: Reis, 2012.

Congenital malformations are one of the main causes of morbidity and mortality in children of mothers with pre-gestational diabetes. High levels of maternal glycaemia or glycohemoglobin during embryogenesis are associated with high rates of spontaneous abortion and major malformations in newborns (LARQUÉ et al., 2014).

The perinatal mortality rate is five times higher in pregnant women with insulin-dependent GDM than in the general population. In order to monitor the vitality of the fetus, fetal monitoring is considered fundamental in such pregnancies, as well as the assessment of fetal growth by ultrasound, FHR monitoring, control of fetal movement, the fetal biophysical profile and dopplervelocimetry of the uterine and fetal circulations (CATALANO;

MOUZON, 2015).

CHAPTER 4

Final considerations

The pathophysiology surrounding gestational diabetes mellitus causes a series of metabolic alterations, leading to a range of maternal and foetal comorbidities. The large amount of glucose in the blood that passes through the placenta into the foetal circulation in GDM gives rise to an abnormal metabolic intrauterine environment and affects the development of the foetus, inducing changes in gene expression through epigenetic mechanisms in susceptible cells, which can lead to the development of diabetes in adulthood.

It was realised that gestational diabetes affects placental homeostasis, and it is therefore necessary to achieve optimal metabolic health before a planned pregnancy, which may offer the best option, and not necessarily the easiest one, to achieve a healthy pregnancy outcome, and eventually within the expected timeframe as well.

As an indispensable member of the multidisciplinary women's and children's health care team, nurses must search for scientific knowledge in this area in order to improve care for this group and monitor the foetus while it is still in the womb, since it can suffer the consequences of this pathology through maternal-placental exchange.

Finally, it can be seen that the objectives set were achieved and this research provides support for interventions for this profile of pregnant women, in order to minimise the occurrence of gestational diabetes mellitus.

This research thus contributes to scientific growth and serves as a future source of consultation for the development of new research, academic teaching and the development of manuals and protocols.

CHAPTER 5

REFERENCES

ABI-ABIB,R.C. et al. DIABETES IN PREGNANCY. HUPE Magazine. v. 13, n.3, p. 4047,2014.

ANTUNES, N de J. et al . Influence of gestational diabetes on the stereoselective pharmacokinetics and placental distribution of metoprolol and its metabolites in parturients. British Journal of Clinical Pharmacology, v.79, n.4, p.605-616, 2015.

ARENDT, L. H.et al. Placental Weight and Male Genital Anomalies: A Nationwide Danish Cohort Study. American Journal of Epidemiology,v.183,n.12,p.112-115,2016.

BAKER, B. C. et al . Placental dysfunction is associated with altered microRNA expression in pregnant women with low folate status. Molecular Nutrition & Food Research, v.61, n.8, p.160-165, 2017.

BORGELT, J.M.A. et al . Assessment of first-trimester thymus size and correlation with maternal diseases and fetal outcome. Acta Obstet Gynecol Scand, v.95, n.8, p.210- 216, 2016.

CATALANO, P; MOUZON, S de. Maternal obesity and metabolic risk to the offspring: why lifestyle interventions may not have achieved the desired outcomes. International journal of obesity, v.39, n.4, p.642-649, 2015.

CATALANO ,P.M. et al. Inadequate weight gain in overweight and obese pregnant women: what is the effect on foetal growth? Am J Obstet Gynecol, v.1, n.7, p.130-137, 2014a.

CATALANO ,P.M. Trying to understand gestational diabetes. Diabetic medicine : a journal of the British Diabetic Association, v.31, n.3, p.273-281, 2014b.

CRUME, T.L. et al. The long-term impact of intrauterine growth restriction in a diverse U.S. cohort of children: the EPOCH study. Obesity, v.22.n.2, p.608-615, 2014.

DESOYE, G.; NOLAN,C. J. The Fetal Glucose Steal: An Underappreciated Phenomenon in Diabetic Pregnancy.Diabetologia 59, v.25, n.6, p.1089-

1094, 2016.

GALVÃO, C.M; SAWADA, N.O; TREVISAN, M.A. Systematic review: a resource for incorporating evidence into nursing practice. Rev Latino-am Enfermagem. v.12, n.3, p. 549-56, mai/jun. 2004.

GIACHINI, F.R.C et al. Maternal Diabetes Affects Specific Extracellular Matrix Components during Placentation.Journal of Anatomy,v.212,n.1,p.31-41,2014.

GIL, A.C. Como elaborar projetos de pesquisa. 4. ed. São Paulo: Atlas, p.174, 2002.

GUILLEMETTE, L. et al. Genetics of Glucose regulation in Gestation and Growth (Gen3G): a prospective prebirth cohort of mother-child pairs in Sherbrooke, Canada. BMJ Open, v.6, n.2, p.530-535, 2016.

GUTAJ, P. et al. Maternal serum placental growth factor and foetal SGA in pregnancy complicated by type 1 diabetes mellitus. Journal of Perinatal Medicine, v.42, n.5, p.629- 633, 2014.

HANTOUSHZADEH, S. et al.The impact of gestational weight gain in different trimesters of pregnancy on glucose challenge test and gestational diabetes. Postgraduate Medical Journal,v.92,n.7,p.520-524,2016.

HE, M. et al.Placental findings associated with maternal obesity at early pregnancy. Pathology - Research and Practice, v.212, n.4, p.282-285, 2016.

HERRERA, E; DESOYE, G.Maternal and foetal lipid metabolism under normal and gestational diabetic conditions. Hormone Molecular Biology and Clinical Investigation, v.26, n.2, p.109-127, 2016.

KAMANA, KC; SHAKYA ,S;ZHANG, H. Gestational Diabetes Mellitus and Macrosomia: A Literature Review. Ann Nutr Metab,v.66, n.2, p.14-20, 2015.

KIM, C. Maternal outcomes and follow-up after gestational diabetes mellitus. Diabetic medicine : a journal of the British Diabetic Association,v.31,n.3,p.292-301,2014.

LARQUÉ, E. et al. Placental Fatty Acid Transfer: A Key Factor in Fetal Growth. Ann Nutr Metab, v.64, n.10, p.247-253, 2014.

LESSEUR, C. et al. Maternal Obesity and Gestational Diabetes are Associated with Placental Leptin DNA Methylation. American journal of obstetrics and gynecology, v.211, n.6.p.12-15, 2014.

LI, G. et al. Early Pregnancy Maternal Lipid Profiles and the Risk of Gestational Diabetes Mellitus Stratified for Body Mass Index. Reproductive Sciences, v.22, n.6, p.712-717, 2015.

LIU, L. et al. Distinct DNA Methylomes of Human Placentas Between Pre-Eclampsia and Gestational Diabetes Mellitus. Cell Physiol Biochem, v.34, n.5, p.1877-1889, 2014.

MARTINO,J. et al. Maternal Body Weight and Gestational Diabetes Differentially Influence Placental and Pregnancy Outcomes. The Journal of Clinical Endocrinology and Metabolism, v.101, n.1, p.59-68, 2016.

MENDES, K.D.S; SILVEIRA, R.C.C.P; GALVÃO, C.M. Revisão Integrativa: Método de Pesquisa para a incorporação de evidências na saúde e na enfermagem. Texto Contexto Enferm, Florianópolis, v.17, n.4,p. 758-64, Oct-Dec, 2008.

REIS, A.R.M dos. Vascular alterations of the placenta and diabetes.Thesis(Integrated Master's Degree in Medicine, scientific area of Obstetrics)- Faculty of Medicine, University of Coimbra.Coimbra,p.12.2012.

ROMANOWSKI, M. et al. Adiponectin and leptin gene polymorphisms in patients with post-transplant diabetes mellitus. Pharmacogenomics. v. 16, n.11, p. 1243-1251, 2015.

SIMONE,N di.et al. Synthetic PreImplantation Factor (PIF) prevents foetal loss by modulating LPS induced inflammatory response. Plos one, v.12, n.7, p.180-187, 2017.

SINGH, A. K.; SINGH, R. Metformin in gestational diabetes: An emerging contender.Indian J Endocrinol Metab, v. 19, n.2, p. 236-44. 2015.

STANEK ,J. Decidual arteriolopathy with or without associated hypertension modifies the underlying histomorphology in placentas from diabetic mothers. Journal of Obstetrics and Gynaecology Research, v.43, n.5, p.839-849, 2017.

STANEK, J;BIESIADA, J.Relation of placental diagnosis in stillbirth to fetal maceration and gestational age at delivery. Journal of Perinatal Medicine, v.42, n.4, p.457-471, 2014.

VRIES, P.S de. et al. Association between polyunsaturated fatty acid concentrations in maternal plasma phospholipids during pregnancy and offspring adiposity at age 7: the MEFAB cohort. Prostaglandins Leukot

Essent Fatty Acids, v.91, n.4, p.81-85, 2014.

ZHANG, Y. et al. Role of high-risk variants in the development of impaired glucose metabolism was modified by birth weight in Han Chinese. Diabetes Metab Res Rev. v. 31, n.8, p. 790-5. 2015.

APPENDIX A

DATA COLLECTION INSTRUMENT	
ARTICLE IDENTIFICATION	
Journal title	
Article title	
Academic background of the author 1 °	
Year of publication	
METHODOLOGICAL CHARACTERISATION OF THE STUDY	
1 Type of study	1.1 Technical procedures ( ) Bibliographical research ( ) Documentary research ( ) Experimental research ( ) Survey ( ) Field study ( ) Case Study ( ) Action research

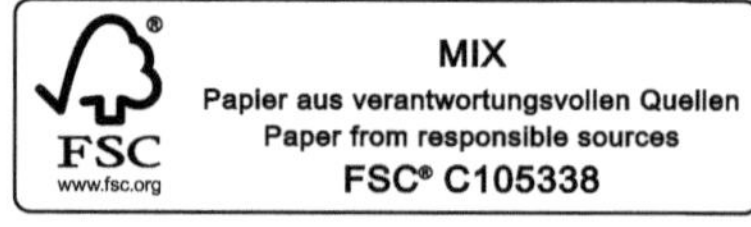

Printed by Books on Demand GmbH, Norderstedt / Germany